CAMPING UNDER THE NIGHT SKY

A meditative story to massage your body
and relax your mind

BOOKS IN THE NATUREBODY® SERIES

—

Walking in an Ancient Forest

Camping Under the Night Sky

Relaxing by a Waterfall

A Peaceful Winter Ski

Swimming in a Tropical Sea

A Healing Coastal Walk

Relaxing in the High Desert

A Spirited Mountain Hike

The complete
NatureBody® Connection
program is available at

www.aquaterramassage.com

A NATUREBODY® MASSAGE STORY

Camping Under the
NIGHT
SKY

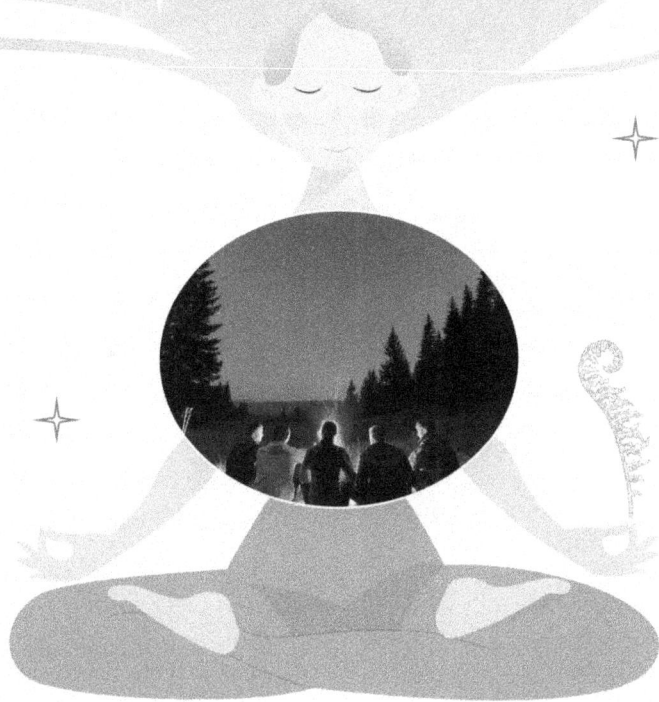

A meditative story to massage your body
and relax your mind

ERIK KRIPPNER *and* FAYE KRIPPNER

ISBN: 978-1-959772-04-0

Cover art provided by Envato Elements. Cover design by Faye Krippner and Erik Krippner.

Release Date for First Printed Edition 2023.

Media Inquiries: If you would like to contact the authors, please send an email to press@aquaterramassage.com.

Faye Krippner, B.A., LMT and Erik Krippner, B.S., LMT have been licensed by the Oregon Board of Massage Therapy since 2003. Oregon License Numbers: 10233 & 10234

Experience the entire NatureBody® Connection at
www.aquaterramassage.com

Dedicated to our ancestors.

Thank you for showing us
that there is more to life
than we see,
and for helping us dream
beyond our boundaries.

Index of Reflections

Contents

How to Use This Book

Humans have lived in balance with our bodies and the earth for 2.6 million years. Our bodies are designed for this planet. It is natural to walk on uneven ground, climb mountains, run long distances, swim, and most of all, to deeply breathe fresh air. Our wild planet heals and strengthens us by making us more flexible and fluid.

Your body is born of this earth. Earth is here to support you. Unfortunately, the stresses of life pull us off balance, and can leave us feeling physically sore and mentally anxious. This creative journey into relaxation is a way to remember your natural balance and create new muscle memories.

As massage therapists, we understand how a relaxed body feels: how it breathes, how it moves, how it is balanced in space. This NatureBody® massage story shares the full spectrum of massage: body, mind and spirit. Our intention is to empower you to find healing within yourself.

Visualization can have powerful effects on your body.[1] In this guided visualization, you will exercise your mind and imagination to deeply relax and bring your body back to center.

If you are injured or your ability to move is limited, then visualization is even more important! Studies have shown that when you imagine moving, the same areas of your brain activate as if you are actually moving those specific muscles.[2] Through visualization, you are virtually exercising your body.

We are intending for you to have a tangible, physical response to the ideas in this book. The power of this story lies in the vividness of your imagination. Read slowly. Pause. Use all of your senses to experience the story. Imagine the changes in humidity. Feel the gentle breeze on your skin. Hear the soothing sound of the wind. Smell the fresh scent of the life around you. Use your vibrant imagination to experience every detail in this story.

Put yourself in the story. Try to experience every sensation in your body. If you feel like moving, do it! Trust your instincts. Imagine what it feels like to move through the story: your muscles warming and stretching... your breathing deepening... your heartbeat slowing as you deeply relax. Let these sensations come to you at the speed of thought. This isn't about concentrating as much as it is about experiencing.

Each time you practice visualizing this story, your experience will become more vibrant. Your body is your wilderness to explore and understand. Your mind is your canvas for new muscle memories.

The Reflections are our personal notes to you. They offer you insight into some of the concepts in the story. Use them to spark your own creative thoughts about connection and healing.

The Notes section is full of wonderful articles and books that we have selected for you. If you feel interested in a topic, we highly recommend you look at the notes to explore the topic further.

The Journal at the end of the book gives you an opportunity to enhance and deepen your meditation. We have asked you a few thought-provoking questions to help you get started. Feel free to write or draw. Journal as creatively as you are inspired. This is your time to dream of the supportive connections between your body and nature.

There is much to discover about your relationship with your body and the beautiful world around you. Find a comfortable place to relax and enjoy. Prepare to be transported to a setting where you can unwind, immersed in nature, and experience the unbridled freedom of the wild!

From Wellness To Oneness,

Erik and Faye
Your Virtual Massage Therapists

FROM WELLNESS TO ONENESS

Wherever you are,

however you feel,

whatever your state of wellness,

know that

healing is at hand.

Your body is always seeking balance

and looking for opportunities to restore.

Through wellness,

may you come to oneness

with your body,

your mind,

your spirit,

and the beautiful Earth that supports us all.

Introduction

Campfires linger in our memories. Jovial evenings with friends around a roaring campfire mellow into the meditative stillness of gazing into the glimmering coals. The stars above encourage us to dream of things greater than ourselves.

This NatureBody® massage story gently guides you to ponder the vastness of the universe

...to meditate with an open heart.

...to exist beyond space and time.

...to be able to be alone, but not lonely.

...to live with your soul, not your skin.

Sit back and let your body unwind as you drift into relaxation, with beautiful visions and deep thoughts under the stars.

To experience the entire

NatureBody® Connection

scan this QR code

or go to

www.aquaterramassage.com / naturebodygift / nightsky

A gift for you, dear reader.

A special reading by the authors awaits you
at the link above.

CHAPTER ONE

Welcome

BREATHING AND THORACIC MASSAGE

W elcome. Come join me by the campfire on this beautiful evening under the stars. Today's hike to this picturesque mountaintop has left my body tired, and my mind clear. My friends and I have built a campfire in a forest clearing and are warming ourselves in its glow. I am deeply enjoying this relaxing evening.

At the edge of the clearing, a spring seeps up out of the rocks. The refreshing mountain water replenishes my reservoir of energy.

The fire is small. It beckons to be enjoyed. It is burning hot and efficiently, and very little smoke comes off of it. Its radiant heat warms the cool evening air. Every once in a while, it crackles. Sparks fly upward, rising to the sky. The rocks underneath the fire glow warmly.

A Relaxing Breath

"My belly rises and falls as I breathe."

One of the things I love best about breathing is that it gives me the opportunity to consciously communicate with my nervous system.

Breathing deep into my abdomen sends signals to my nervous system to relax. In this relaxed state, my body dispels the chemicals of anxiety and brings me into a state of well being. Through breathing, I can move out of the anxious, fight-or-flight response and into the healing, rest-and-digest state.[3] I am communicating with my nervous system that "all is well."

Standing or sitting tall, feel your breath lower into your abdomen. Take your time with your exhale. Empty all the air out of your lungs. Let your inhale come naturally and quietly.

It may help to visualize what is happening internally. Your diaphragm is an dome-shaped muscle. When it contracts, it flattens downward, opening your lungs. This creates a vacuum that draws in air. As your diaphragm lowers, your abdominal organs shift downward to make space.

Breathing in and out, your organs lower and rise in an undulating motion, as if they were being gently massaged. This rhythmic motion helps the flow of your digestion.[4]

Through this simple pattern of breathing, you are guiding your body into a healing state of being.

Our view of the sky is crystal clear down to the tree-lined horizon. I am breathing pure mountain air on this beautiful evening.

I begin to center and relax.

Breathing in, I feel my belly expand.

I let it fall as I breathe out.

On my next inhale,
    I imagine my breath
    entering through my belly button.

Now, as I exhale,
    very lightly,
    I engage my abdominal muscles.

I keep my abs engaged slightly as I breathe in,
    letting my lower ribcage widen.

I exhale without resistance.

My belly rises and falls
    as I breathe.

When I take my next inhale, I imagine the air could fill my back as much as it did my belly.

The back of my ribs expand away from my spine.

My torso becomes wider.

Breathing for a Healthy Low Back

"My breath has found its foundation at the base of my pelvis."

Breathing is a great way to maintain a supple, elastic pelvic floor.[5] A healthy pelvic floor dynamically stabilizes our low back when we walk or run, stand or sit. It also supports our pelvic organs and their functions. As you inhale and exhale, your pelvic floor naturally expands and contracts. Breathing is essential to our pelvic floor health.

When you breathe low into your lungs (diaphragmatic breathing) your diaphragm lowers, pressing your abdominal contents down toward your pelvis. Your pelvic floor muscles respond by stretching to allow space.[6] When you exhale, your pelvic floor muscles return to their toned position. Incorporating your pelvis in your breathing makes you more efficient during athletic performance, more relaxed, and more physically balanced.

Let's try an exercise to breathe fully, down to your pelvic floor. Lightly engage your abdominal muscles and inhale. Feel your breath sink all the way down the column of your spine into your hips. Don't let your ribs flare or your belly spill out. Keep drawing your breath downward. Imagine your pelvic floor expanding to make room for your inhale.

Exhale fully, squeezing the air out of your lungs. Finish your exhale by gently contracting your pelvic floor[7] and your abdominal muscles. Relax your pelvic floor on your next inhale. This is an effective way to maintain the healthy tone of your pelvic floor muscles. You are breathing with your whole being.

Soft throat.

Broad chest.

I let the extra effort spill lower,
*   down to the tops of my legs.*

I imagine my heels are reaching,
*   filling with air.*

The backs of my legs become longer.

My breath has found its foundation
*   at the base of my pelvis.*

As I find my breath
*   lower and lower in my body,*
*   my shoulders drop,*
*   my chest relaxes*
*   and my throat softens.*

My breath is now flowing
*   along my whole body,*
*   from my perineum*
*   to the crown of my head.*

The energy of my breath
*   stokes my center,*
*   and shines out my fingers and toes.*

Energetic Flow

"I AM the flow."

In Eastern medicine, a healthy body depends on the steady flow of life energy, or "chi," through the body.[8]

Chi flows through the yin meridians up the front and inside of your body. It returns downward through the yang channels on the back and outside of your body.

Imagine breathing with this flow of chi in mind.

As you inhale, imagine a narrow stream of powerful energy flowing upward along your midline (yin). Draw energy up through your feet. Feel it rising up the center of your body. It flows narrowly up the inside of your legs, your pelvis, your abdomen, your throat, and up to the crown of your head. Picture that energy transforming into the strength your body needs to rise tall through gravity.

When you exhale, visualize a waterfall of relaxed energy cascading down the outside (yang) of your body. Imagine the energy flowing down your back and the outside of your arms and legs, and back into the ground. Let this flow encourage your limbs to be free, flexible, and ready for action.

The postural reach of my breath
    is like a fountain.

It flows from the soles of my feet,
    up my midline,
    to the crown of my head.

The return flow
    relaxes any extra muscular effort,
    like a waterfall,
    down my shoulders,
    my arms,
    my outer legs
    to my feet.

My body feels long and flowing.

I feel the flow,
    the rising narrow fountain of my inhale,
    the plunging broad waterfall of my exhale.

I AM the flow.

CHAPTER TWO

The Evening Deepens

QUIETING THE MIND

W e are gathered in a clearing in an evergreen forest on this cool summer night. The campfire has burned down to a warm glow. My friends and I move a little closer to the fire.

Earlier, the fire danced and sparks launched upwards. We talked through the evening, laughing together and sharing stories of our adventures. The evening matured and the sky darkened. Sunset transformed into twilight. The evening star, Venus, rose brilliantly in the east. The sky continued to deepen into a rich sapphire. Inky silhouettes of fir trees outline the horizon.

We look up into the velvet black sky. One by one, stars appear, until the sky is sprinkled with millions. Strewn with innumerable stars, the night sky guides our minds away from any remaining thought into the awe of our humble place in this vast universe, in this present moment.

Your Inner Fire

*"The pulsing heat through the carbon of the coals
reflects the life-force pulsing through the carbon of my body."*

The Earth's molten core is liquid fire. This swirling, liquid iron provides the electric energy that gives Earth its magnetic charge.[9]

Your body also has its own electrical charge from the vibration of your living cells. Your cells vibrate and generate an electrical current like Earth's magnetosphere.[10] You are an energetic being.

You strengthen your energy through breath[11] and movement.[12] When you breathe, exhale completely. Allow your lungs to empty. Pause in this moment of stillness. Inhale through your nose: a fresh, energizing breath that warms the air as it spirals through your sinuses.

Movement and breathing are catalysts for change. Motion heats your muscles, helping them to become both stronger and more flexible. Whether you move slowly or quickly, a lot or a little, keep moving. Your body is designed to move.

Breath and movement kindle your inner fire and add vitality to the energetic vibration of your body.

My friends and I are silent now. The warmth of the fire draws our gaze back to its glowing red embers. Circled around the campfire, we warm our hands in its radiant glow.

The fire crackles faintly. The glow of the coals pulses as if living bands of heat are traveling through them.

> *The pulsing heat through the carbon of the coals*
> *reflects the life-force pulsing through*
> *the carbon of my body.*

> *The fire mesmerizes me.*

A friend uses the fire poker to gather the coals together. A shower of sparks floats up, and disappears into the stars. We move a little closer to the fire. As it dwindles, I feel the chill of the evening curl up against my back.

The gathering is beginning to wind down. Some of my companions have already slipped away into their sleeping bags. The growing cool wraps around me, inspiring me to make the primal effort of moving to my final shelter for the night. I stand tall, stir the fire one last time and gaze at its glowing red galaxy of embers. Absolute blackness fills the gaps between the radiant red-hot coals.

I tell my friends goodnight, and amble just a few feet away to the other side of the tree where I had set up my bedroll. I climb into my sleeping bag and gaze up through the sparse branches to the stars above. A blanket of stars shimmers above me.

> *I stare dreamily into the night sky,*
> *and relax deeply.*

CHAPTER THREE

Cohesiveness in Space: Filling the Void

SOOTHING THE NERVOUS SYSTEM

M y friends have already started to doze nearby. I can hear their restful breathing. My bedroll lies under an evergreen tree, whose coniferous scent freshens the mountain air. I look forward to dreaming under its wisdom.

This tree's craggy form helps define the character of its life. It has seen many centuries pass. Strong winds have pruned its fine branches. Only strong, sinewy branches remain facing the wind. There are more fine branches on the other side of the tree, protected in the safety of the forest.

Over the years, a thick bed of evergreen needles has collected under the tree. Nature has designed them to burn hot and keep the tree's neighbors well spaced. The soft needles under the tree make a comfortable bed for slumber.

On Space

"The vacuum of space felt cold and lifeless, infinitely devoid of warmth and comfort."

The darkness between stars... The silence between sounds... The stillness between breaths...

I associate space with a pure, clear mind. Life, for all its beauty and color, is energy. Although you can't visually see it, your energy is just as animated as all the colors of the rainbow. That is what I see in space.

Even on a physical level, we are mostly space. If the nucleus of one of your atoms was the size of an orange, an electron in that same atom would be the size of a grain of sand... over a mile away! Vast tracts of space fill us at an atomic level, even though our bodies feel solid and tactile.[13]

Acknowledging the energy all around us fills the void, and brings hope and comfort to even the bleakest of thoughts. To know you are surrounded by, and part of, a supportive energy that is always present, is to know you are never alone.

I slide into my sleeping bag, pulling the pillowy, silky fabric up around my shoulders. My sleeping bag is roomy, wide enough for me to spread out. I feel delightfully warm as my body rests into the cushion of soft, evergreen needles.

The clear night is inviting. It is cool outside, but not cold. I am lying under a tapestry of stars.

My breathing effortlessly fills my center,
*   allowing my legs to reach long and relax.*

My arms rest naturally at my sides.

I breathe the heaviness out of my low back.

My spine grows longer as I inhale
*   and feels more supported as I exhale.*

The blackness above becomes thicker, richer, and the stars shimmer. As night deepens, the Milky Way slowly reveals itself. The sky is now an inky black. The galaxy is spectacular: a thick cloud of billions of stars.

I am looking into the center of our spiraling galaxy.

In the winter, the Milky Way seems much smaller and fainter. In that season, we are looking outward, beyond the disc of our galaxy, into the outer reaches of space.

Now, in the summer, we are oriented so that we look toward the billions of stars in the heart of our galaxy. There are a few dark spots in this galactic cloud: spaces between the stars where I see into deep space.

Visualize to Realize

---

*"A wavelike action of electrons
fills the emptiness with their potential..."*

As science continues to discover more about our universe,
we have come to understand that energy and matter are
intimately related. From Einstein's theory of relativity[14] to
quantum physics,[15] modern science shows that energy can
behave like matter, and matter, like energy.

Since your physical body has qualities of both energy and
matter, you can use one to influence the other. You can use
the energy of thought to influence the "matter" of your
body. *Thinking differently helps you change.*

Visualization is a powerful way to use the electricity of
your mind to create new pathways in your brain. The same
areas of your prefrontal cortex light up whether you are
physically moving or thinking of moving. Your brain does
not distinguish between physical action and imagination.[16]

You can use visualization to manage stress, boost your
immune system, and improve athletic performance. The
more vividly you imagine, using all your senses, the more
effective visualization becomes. As you focus your
thoughts, your brain looks for ways to make them true.[17]
Let yourself see, smell, hear, touch and even taste the
reality you want to create.

You are energetically paving the way to physically become
what you visualize.

Deep space... we first assumed it was a vast emptiness with everything hurtling farther away, still surfing on the push of the big bang. I used to feel lonely thinking of the accelerating void between ourselves and all other planets, stars, and potential life. The vacuum of space felt cold and lifeless, infinitely devoid of warmth and comfort. But the concept of dark matter changed the way I felt.

We haven't tangibly detected dark matter. But when you include the concept of dark matter in our understanding of the universe, suddenly our universal understanding is more complete. Dark matter fills the void of space. It fortifies the cohesiveness of our universe: the gathering and spinning of solar systems and galaxies.[18]

I am comforted by the idea
    that there is no void,
    no immeasurable emptiness.

Instead,
    something intangible,
    something mysterious,
    surrounds and infuses every space.

My body is a product of the universe.

As I relate to the space that surrounds me,
    I am compelled to entertain the space that fills me.
    A space that on an atomic level,
    is every bit as sparse as the universe.

My body is almost entirely space.
    It is connected more by energy
    than by the solid mass I perceive.

Healing Potential

"My body is a framework for the flow of life to exist in me."

You are more like a wave of energy than a solid, unchanging particle. Because it is in our nature to be fluid and constantly changing, healing is not only possible, but likely.

In our massage practice, we have seen many people pleasantly surprised by how much relief they feel from their massage. Aches and pains they were convinced were permanent, changed, and sometimes quietly disappeared. It is our fluid, wavelike nature that makes massaging our particles so powerfully effective.

Our bodies are always looking for balance. The more we nurture our bodies and minds, the more our bodies are able to perform, and the more we can maintain a healthy state of mind. This positive feedback loop is a cornerstone to healing. Positive input like water, food, sleep, and exercise creates more positive outcomes. It is not so much that our bodies are machines to be driven, as they are vessels to be nourished and nurtured.

When you feel stuck or stagnant, remember the fluid, wavelike nature of your body. Your body is poised to respond to changing conditions. Drink water. Move your body. Eat nourishing food. Breathe.

Give your body the opportunity to heal. Allow your light to shine.

The void within me is filled with a smear of energy. A wavelike action of electrons fills the emptiness with their potential to exist at any given point... at any given moment. With almost no mass at all, electrons fill the space within me with their trembling, wavelike nature.

> As an electron behaves both as a particle and a wave,
>   so do I share in this understanding
>   that though I exist as a physical human,
>   I have always been connected
>   to the boundless energy of the universe.

> My body is a framework
>   for the flow of life
>   to exist in me.

> There is a pattern,
>   a beautiful symmetry to everything.

> I am an antenna for the universe.

CHAPTER FOUR

The Galactic Show

CRANIAL AND JAW MASSAGE

I am warm and cozy in my sleeping bag. The cool night air blows gently across my face. The crickets are starting to sing and the soundscape becomes as full as the starry sky. The splendid spectacle of this galactic show excites my imagination.

The stars tell of their history in our present, as their light which reaches my eye now, is as old as the star is distant: light years away. The rich night sky tells an ancient story.

Our ancestors gazed upon the same stars I dreamily contemplate now. I look for familiar constellations, greeting them like old friends.

I always notice the Big Dipper first. I follow the far side of its ladle up to find Polaris, the North Star, whose dependable position, together with the Southern Cross, marks Earth's pirouette along the celestial plane.

On Peripheral Vision

"I open my eyes to see everything that is around me."

As a forester, I spent a lot of time walking while looking up at trees. I used my peripheral vision to stay aware of what was around me while I focused on the trees. My peripheral vision kept me from falling.

Learning to use our peripheral vision helps our balance. It can prevent us from becoming tunnel visioned or point fixated. Paying attention to what is going on in our periphery makes us more mindful of where we are in space.

Try this exercise to strengthen your eyes and develop your peripheral vision.

Just using your eyes, look to the right, left, up and down. Next, follow your eye movements with your head. (For example, look to the right, then turn your head to the right.) Create space in your neck by lowering your shoulders and reaching tall out of the crown of your head. Focus on your long spine and level vision.

Gaze forward, stretch your arms out to the sides, and wiggle your fingertips. Without moving your head or eyes, try to see your fingertips in your periphery. This shows you the edges of your peripheral vision.

Peripheral vision invites us to become aware of, and connected to, the world around us.[19]

Orion's belt glints as he holds a strong posture, sword at his side. He is magnificent in his presence. And there is the familiar "W" shape of Cassiopeia, the regal queen who sits eternally upon her golden throne.

The stars appear to twinkle as they shine through the shimmery veil of Earth's atmosphere. Some stars are so faint that I cannot see them when I look directly at them. They are only visible in my peripheral vision.

It is fun to play with my peripheral vision. I look directly at a star and it disappears. I look away, and it reappears in the side of my vision.

I open my eyes to see everything that is around me.

I see to the edges of my gaze,
aware of everything to the right and left,
up and down.

My head sinks back into the sleeping bag
and my neck releases.

The muscles at the base of my skull open.

My throat softens.
My tongue relaxes.
Even my teeth feel like they relax.

I breathe
and imagine space in my head,
as if my brain is expanding.

There is a swirling galaxy inside my head.

Listening to Silence

"My ears reach to detect the soft sounds of the now silent night."

Silence is a unique vibration.

When we finally come out of the noise of the world, we hear a ringing as sounds dissipate from our heads. The tympanic membrane and the hairlike cilia in our ears return to stillness; returning to silence.

As you strive to be more sensitive to sound, notice your body responding. Your breathing quiets. Your neck muscles lengthen to be more receptive. The temporal muscles under your ears feel like they reach to detect sound.

Become aware of the quiet vibration of the world around you. You can hear
...the inner workings of your body.
...the hushed whisper of your breathing.
...the gurgling of your stomach.
...the flow of your circulation.
...the drum of your heartbeat.

Silence is never truly "silent." Quiet provides an opportunity for us to listen deeper.

My ears reach to detect
    the soft sounds of the now silent night.

The drumbeat of my heart
    brings rhythm to the night sky.

I close my eyes and watch the light dissipate
    as the energy of my brain
    finishes sending the signals
    it has already received.

I imagine the air is heavy.

I inhale, and
    drink the air down the back of my body,
    expanding
    my connection with the earth.

I exhale effortlessly.

I inhale.
    The air flows into my mid-back
    and then sinks down into my hips.

I exhale.
    I feel the spirit of the previous breath
    infusing my cells.

I inhale.
    My body is opening and expanding,
    dissolving into space
    beyond my skin.

"Our Space"

"My space is spoken for. Our space is yet to be revealed."

On an energetic level, there is no time or space. We come from energy and we return to energy. The vibration we leave is timeless. It is the expression of our matter that emits energy into the universe.

Our "matter" is our physical body. We express our "energy" through our actions, our movement, and breathing. Pursuing health brings an intention to our vibration.

Striving to be healthier and more balanced, sends a ripple of energy through the universe. A wave of love, health, compassion, and empathy emanates from your thriving body.

Just as dark energy accelerates the expansion of the universe, this loving, healing energy continually grows. Love is a catalyst for begetting more: more love, more understanding, and more healing.

Sharing your loving energy helps others find it in themselves. A ripple builds into a wave, creating a critical mass of healing energy that reaches a tipping point, leading to a paradigm shift in understanding.[20]

The vibration each of us emits is our eternal ripple in this beautiful pond. Our collective ripples combine into the fabric of this vast and precious universal sea of energy.

I exhale,
  and return to the peace of possibility.

My awareness reaches beyond my conscious understanding,
  beyond this mountain clearing,
  beyond the galactic reaches of the Milky Way,
  to the very edges of the universe.

But, what lies beyond?

My space is spoken for.
  Our space is yet to be revealed.

What possibilities of communion with the cosmos can you imagine?

Dream on, Tranquil Wanderer.

CHAPTER FIVE

The Cosmic Dance

GROUNDING AND POSTURAL RELEASE

E xcept for three star clusters, everything we can see with our naked eye resides in our galaxy. There are billions of stars in the Milky Way, our galactic home.

How many planets with each of these stars?
How many moons with each of these planets?

The orbital dance of our solar system joins the cosmic dance of other celestial bodies, all swirling around a massive black hole in the center of the Milky Way.

It is as if everything is part of a grand design:
    dancing,
    swirling,
    connected by energy.

You Belong

"I am a part of the dance of the stars."

The protons and neutrons that make up the atoms in your body were created one second after the Big Bang. They have existed for over 13.7 billion years. Most of the elements in your body were created within stars. You are formed from stardust.[21]

On an energetic level, your body and mind emit energy, making you an energetic being.[22] The molecules in your body vibrate at different rates, and can speed up or slow down to react to the changing conditions around them.[23] Your heart, brain, hormones and nervous system all respond to music.[24] Your body vibrates and creates energy.

There is so much more to you than what seems to exist on the surface.

You are related to the stars. When you focus your awareness on the physical and energetic being that you are, you can sense your pure belonging in this universe.

As one of life's miracles, you are exactly where you are supposed to be.

Here, in the center of my sleeping bag,
*   I project my awareness outward,*
*   feeling that there is no earth beneath me.*

That I am, in fact, floating in space.
*   Exactly where I am supposed to be.*

I am a part of the dance of the stars.

I belong to the earth,
*   the stars,*
*   the universe.*

The atoms that make me, have been here since time began. I am made of stardust, of planetary elements, forged from the cooling ylem[25] of the Big Bang. The building blocks of my body have existed since less than one second after time began.

*   I am boundless.*

As nourishment enters and leaves my body, I am continually renewing the atoms of which my body is comprised. How I renew my body with energy, and how I spend that energy, is my communication with the universe.

*   It is as if the universe is speaking with me.*

*   I have been created as the perfect antenna*
*   to receive this universal energy*
*   and to express it through my love and creativity.*

On Posture and Presence

*"I am now a being aware of what is inside of me,
what is behind me, what is around me."*

Our posture can influence our outlook. When we focus forward, paying attention to what is happening in front of us, we tend to jut our chins forward, as if we are keeping our "eyes on the goal." This pulls our heavy heads forward off our center of gravity. Our neck muscles compensate by tightening to hold our head up. The shape of this posture is like the turbulent foam of a cresting wave, falling over itself. It is as if we are leading with our heads into the future.

We can use our posture to help bring ourselves back into the present moment. Try this exercise.

Soften and level your gaze. Become aware of your periphery. Bring your head back over your spine. Feel your neck muscles adjust as they welcome this new posture. Balance yourself by bringing your awareness down to your center of gravity: the Sea of Chi[26] acupressure point just below your navel. Let your breathing become full and satisfying.

As you do this exercise, your awareness naturally shifts. You transition from "doing" and relax into "being." You are becoming a receiver of energy, aware of what is around you and within you.

As you bring your head home over your center of gravity, you are more like a balanced, smooth wave, no longer cresting into the future. Think of your energy as an ocean swell: calm and powerful. You are a full presence of energy.

The stars are shadowed as an owl glides silently
overhead and perches in a tree nearby. I wait to hear for his
call, but he is silent.

The fire is glowing in the distance and a couple of friends are
still sitting near it. My body stretches comfortably in my
sleeping bag. I feel the smooth material slide past my arm as
I move.

I close my eyes
    and imagine a million stars in my body.

My peripheral awareness
    expands to infinity within me.

I am no longer a forward-propelling human,
    focused on what is in front of me.

I am now a being
    aware of what is inside of me,
    what is behind me,
    what is around me.

I imagine looking out at the world
    from the back of my neck.

The muscles at the base of my skull expand and soften.

My jaw loosens
    and I feel an expansiveness in my shoulders,
    my ribs,
    and down my spine
    to my low back and hips.

The Pause Between Breaths

"Between the exhale and the next inhale,
I am deeply connected to spirit."

We are always engaged in the fluid act of breathing. Through breath, we are intimately connected in the flow of life.

It has been said that we are most connected to spirit between the exhale and the inhale, when our lungs are empty.[27]

Draw out your next exhale. Pause at the end.

The space between breaths is a moment of presence and awareness.

It is a moment of stillness. A moment of faith.

Now inhale the first breath of the rest of your life!

This spacious release
  floods down into my sacrum,
  my tailbone,
  my legs and my feet.

I inhale,
  and then I exhale,
  holding my breath out for a few seconds.

Between the exhale
  and the next inhale,
  I am deeply connected to spirit.

This is the moment of surrender, of mortality: the place where I put my trust into my higher power. Trust that the next breath will come... and that someday, it won't. Yet I am always held in the embrace of purity, symmetry, and perfection of all that surrounds me.

My next inhale tingles with life. I revel in being.

I exhale a swirling vortex of atoms,
  picturing them float up
  and blend into the stars above.

The fog of my exhale in the cool night air
  dissolves into the cloud of our Milky Way.

I blend into
  ...the earth
  ...the sky
  ...space
  becoming part of the timeless universe.

THE COSMIC DANCE

CHAPTER SIX

Gratitude

BLESSING OF THE COSMOS

T hank you for joining me. Since the dawn of time, humans have spent long evenings contemplating the night sky, finding connection and meaning in the stars above.

May the strength of the sun
charge the aura of your being.

May the soft light of the moon
fill the Sea of Tranquility in your soul.

May you find inspiration in the stars,
like bright new ideas born from remnants of the past.

May the swirling dance of our galaxy envelop you
  in the joy of belonging
  in this magnificent universe.

Float on, Tranquil Wanderer. May we meet again in some other space and time.

Acknowledgments

The ideas in this story have come to us over the last few decades. We have enjoyed the study of, and many meditations on our universe and our place in it.

I began my fascination with the stars on a boy scout trip. I still remember sleeping under the stars and waking up with a layer of frost on my sleeping bag. I am grateful to the scouts for introducing me to many amazing experiences.

Thanks to Taylor Sims for studying the planisphere with me on a mushroom-shaped rock in the middle of Canyonlands National Park in Utah. That night has helped me keep my stargazing bearings ever since.

Faye and I thoroughly enjoyed Troy Carpenter's wonderfully engaging talks at the Goldendale Space Observatory in Washington state. Troy described the stars in a way that brought the night sky to life. (If you get a chance to visit Goldendale, consider attending one of Troy's talks!)

Our cousin Douglas, who conducts particles at nearly the speed of light, inspires us with his efforts to bring healing to those who are striving for life.

We deeply appreciated the NOVA documentary, *The Elegant Universe*. Professor Brian Greene's clear explanation of theoretical physics was captivating and easy to understand.

We are grateful to fellow Eagle Scout, our uncle Dr. Randy Bollinger, for his wonderful family bonfires. Stories and songs were shared in camaraderie around the fires in his backyard. Randy's sensitive speech and healing touch has inspired us and our massage palpation throughout our careers. It is in thanks to you, Randy, that we hold up our mugs for another Good Ol' Mountain Dew!

ACKNOWLEDGMENTS

Notes

1. "What is Imagery?" *Johns Hopkins Medicine*, 2003, www.hopkinsmedicine.org/health/wellness-and-prevention/imagery.

2. Lohr, Jim. "Can Visualizing Your Body Doing Something Help You Learn to Do It Better?" *Scientific American*, 1 May 2015, www.scientificamerican.com/article/can-visualizing-your-body-doing-something-help-you-learn-to-do-it-better.

3. "Your Parasympathetic Nervous System Explained." *Healthline*, 2022, www.healthline.com/health/parasympathetic-nervous-system.

4. "Diaphragmatic Breathing for GI Patients." *University of Michigan Health*, 2022, www.uofmhealth.org/conditions-treatments/digestive-and-liver-health/diaphragmatic-breathing-gi-patients.

5. "Pelvic Floor Muscles." *Cleveland Clinic*, 2022, my.clevelandclinic.org/health/body/22729-pelvic-floor-muscles.

6. Patrick, M., & Keesee, J. "Part I: Breathing Techniques for Pelvic Floor Health." *Pelvic Health & Rehabilitation Center*, 2022, pelvicpainrehab.com/pelvic-floor-yoga-and-pilates/18519/part-i-breathing-techniques-for-pelvic-floor-health.

7. Olsen, Amanda. "Proper Kegel Breathing Techniques for Kegel Exercises." *Intimate Rose*, 2023, www.intimaterose.com/blogs/videos/kegel-breathing.

8. Williams, Tom. *Chinese Medicine: Acupuncture, Herbal Remedies, Nutrition, Qigong & Meditation for Total Health*, Massachusetts: Element Books, 1995, pp. 33-42.

9. "How Does the Earth's Core Generate a Magnetic Field?" *USGS*, www.usgs.gov/faqs/how-does-earths-core-generate-magnetic-field. Accessed on 18 January 2023.

10. Plante, Amber. "How the Human Body Uses Electricity." *University of Maryland Graduate Studies*, February 2016, graduate.umaryland.edu/gsa/gazette/February-2016/How-the-human-body-uses-electricity.

11. Burgin, Timothy. "7 Morning Breathing Exercises to Boost Energy and Productivity." *Yoga Basics*, www.yogabasics.com/practice/pranayama/morning-breathing-exercises. Accessed 25 February 2023.

12. Golin, T. and Ricoletti, H. "Does Exercise Really Increase Energy Levels?" *Harvard Health Publishing Harvard Medical School*, 1 July 2021, www.health.harvard.edu/exercise-and-fitness/does-exercise-really-boost-energy-levels.

13. Sundermier, A. "99.9999999% of Your Body Is Empty Space." *Science Alert*, 23 September 2016, www.sciencealert.com/99-9999999-of-your-body-is-empty-space.

14. "Energy." *American Museum of Natural History,* www.amnh.org/exhibitions/einstein/energy. Accessed 18 January 2023.

15. Zimmerman Jones, Andrew. "Wave Particle Duality and How It Works." *ThoughtCo,* 3 July 2019, www.thoughtco.com/wave-particle-duality-2699037.

16. Zlatopolsky, Ashley. "How To Destress with Calming Pictures." *Health,* 2 November 2022, www.health.com/condition/stress/relaxing-images-to-destress.

17. Pax, Prakash Joshi. "The Reticular Activating System and Goal Setting." *Medium,* 6 January 2021, medium.com/change-your-mind/the-reticular-activating-system-and-goal-setting-954fa103024e.

18. "What is Dark Matter?" *NASA,* 22 February 2012, www.nasa.gov/audience/forstudents/9-12/features/what-is-dark-matter.html.

19. Goldstein, William. "A Guide to Understanding Your Peripheral Vision." *Eye Health Web,* February 2016, www.eyehealthweb.com/peripheral-vision.

20. "The Tipping Point by Malcolm Gladwell." *What You Will Learn,* www.whatyouwilllearn.com/book/the-tipping-point-malcolm-gladwell-behaviour. Accessed 18 January 2023.

21. Lotzof, Kerry. "Are We Really Made of Stardust?" *National History Museum,* www.nhm.ac.uk/discover/are-we-really-made-of-stardust.html. Accessed 13 January 2023.

22. Layton, Julia and Mancini, M. "How Does the Body Make Electricity? And How Does It Use It?" *How Stuff Works,* 1 August 2022, health.howstuffworks.com/human-body/systems/nervous-system/human-body-make-electricity.htm.

23. Stanborough, Rebecca. "What Is Vibrational Energy?" *Healthline*, 13 November 2020, www.healthline.com/health/vibrational-energy.

24. Muehsam, David, and Carlo Ventura. "Life Rhythm as a Symphony of Oscillatory Patterns: Electromagnetic Energy and Sound Vibration Modulates Gene Expression for Biological Signaling and Healing." *Global Advances In Health and Medicine*, vol. 3, no. 2, 2014, pp. 40-55. doi:10.7453/gahmj.2014.008.

25. "Ylem" is thought to be the original primordial matter of the universe from which all subatomic particles and elements were formed. "Ylem." *Merriam-Webster Dictionary*, www.merriam-webster.com/dictionary/ylem. Accessed 20 January 2023.

26. Sea of Qi, is an acupressure point located 1.5 inches below the navel. It is considered to be the reservoir of life force. For information, see Beinfeld, Harriet and Korngold, Efrem. *Between Heaven and Earth: A Guide to Chinese Medicine.* New York: Ballentine Publishing Group, 1991, pp. 198.

27. Quam, Christine. "Kumbhaka: The Power of the Pause." *Green Lotus Yoga and Healing Center,* www.greenlotusyogactr.com/nutrition-health-wellness/the-power-of-pause. Accessed 6 February 2023.

MEDITATION

Journal

This journal gives you a place to reflect on your experience as you read and meditate. With every meditation, your library of personal affirmations can grow. Some thoughts you might want to record, in words or drawings, are:

What were your favorite phrases or ideas in the story?

Describe your evening at the campfire. What feelings, energies, or people were present at your campfire to make it feel safe, warm, fun, and complete?

This meditation primarily focused on your head, neck, and jaw. What physical sensations did you notice in your body before, during and after the meditation? How did your breathing change?

Write about wonder, miracles, and love. How do you see yourself as a conduit of love in the universe?

"I BELONG TO THE EARTH, THE
STARS, THE UNIVERSE."

MEDITATION

The components of your body have existed since the beginning of time. You have been stardust. You have been part of galactic winds. Your particles have settled on this planet... in this body... for your expression of life.

You are life, flowing through this beautiful universe.

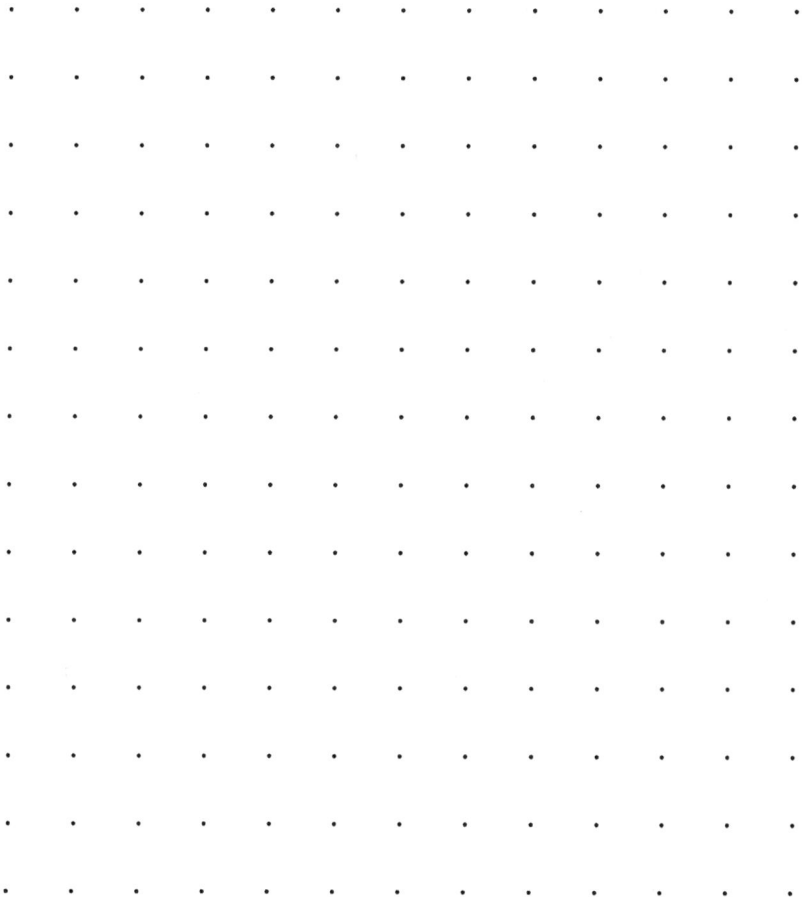

~

"I EXHALE, AND RETURN TO THE
PEACE OF POSSIBILITY."

MEDITATION

Consider what you would like to invite into your life. Exhale. Focus on this thought, and savor your next inhale.

~

May the

STRENGTH

of the

SUN

charge the aura

of your being.

"OUR ANCESTORS GAZED UPON
THE SAME STARS I DREAMILY
CONTEMPLATE NOW. I LOOK FOR
FAMILIAR CONSTELLATIONS,
GREETING THEM LIKE OLD
FRIENDS."

MEDITATION

Our ancient DNA has been passed down through the generations. You have inherited your genetic imprint from your ancestors. Written in every cell is the eons-old story of your legacy.

Long before your DNA was formed, the elements that comprise you were born with the galaxy. You are made of stardust. You are intrinsically connected to your ancestors and the universe: a bond that transcends time and space.

~

"THE EVENING MATURED AND
THE SKY DARKENED. SUNSET
TRANSFORMED INTO TWILIGHT."

MEDITATION

At the closing of each day, twilight arrives. Every sunset invites us to let evening's calm into our bodies. Twilight is a peaceful time to reflect.

Immerse yourself in the waning light and embrace the coming peace of nighttime.

~

May the

SOFT LIGHT

of the

MOON

fill the

Sea of Tranquility

in your soul.

"STREWN WITH INNUMERABLE STARS, THE NIGHT SKY GUIDES OUR MINDS AWAY FROM ANY REMAINING THOUGHT INTO THE AWE OF OUR HUMBLE PLACE IN THIS VAST UNIVERSE, IN THIS PRESENT MOMENT."

MEDITATION

There is an understanding that is deeper than thought: a moment when you understand something so well, that it grows beyond logic, language, and reason, into a full-body knowing. Your body's awareness is infinitely more perceptive than your awareness of your body. Your body's wisdom runs deep.

The meditative mind is not distracted by thoughts or theory. It is naturally focused in being-ness. By being present, we evolve through human *doing*, into human *being*.

~

"THERE IS A PATTERN: A
BEAUTIFUL SYMMETRY TO
EVERYTHING."

MEDITATION

Yʘou are part of nature's design. You are one with the harmonious geometry of the planet. As you reflect on your body, can you see the patterns of nature?

~

May you find

INSPIRATION

in the

STARS

like bright new ideas

born from remnants

of the past.

"ABSOLUTE BLACKNESS FILLS
THE GAPS BETWEEN THE RADIANT
RED-HOT COALS."

MEDITATION

Color fills our beautiful world. We look around and there is a visual feast for our eyes. Our eyes are drawn to the wavelengths of color. Yet, non-color, or absolute blackness, is also mesmerizing. Pure darkness speaks of the presence of a different kind of energy.

We look *at* color: we can look *into* blackness. Allow your eyes to relax in the darkness. Feel your vision shift as you gaze into black. Let your thoughts come and go as you allow your eyes to experience non-light.

Color is energy. Energy is perpetual and continuous. Wherever you look, however you see, you resonate with the omnipresent energy of the universe.

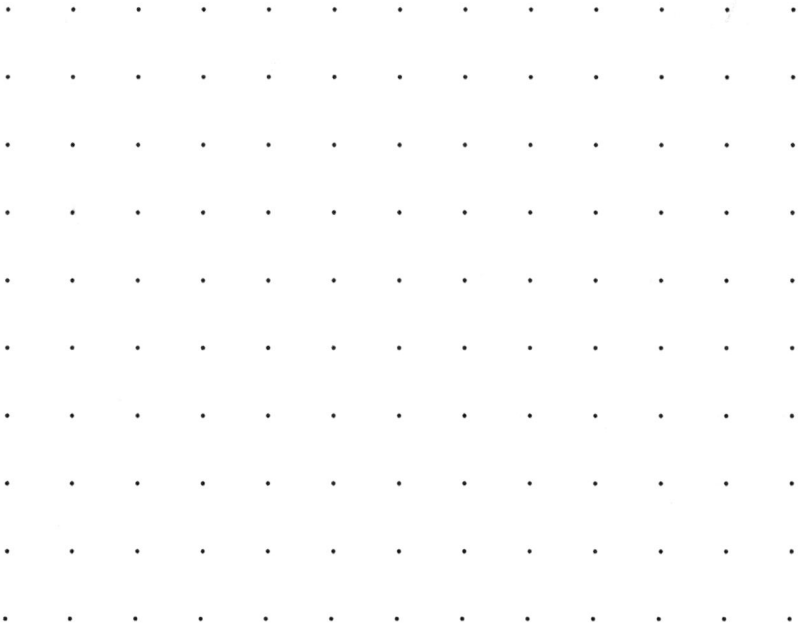

~

"I WILL ALWAYS BE HELD IN THE
EMBRACE OF PURITY, SYMMETRY,
AND PERFECTION OF ALL THAT
SURROUNDS ME."

MEDITATION

The earth is full of beauty and wonder. Even the simplest of things has a unique brilliance: a crescent moon, a flower in full bloom, or a leaf that has drifted down to the ground. There is a season and a time for all things. In this perfection, you belong.

~

May the

SWIRLING

DANCE

of our

GALAXY

envelop you in

the joy of belonging

in this

magnificent universe.

"THIS TREE'S CRAGGY FORM HELPS DEFINE THE CHARACTER OF ITS LIFE. IT HAS SEEN MANY CENTURIES PASS. STRONG WINDS HAVE PRUNED ITS FINE BRANCHES. ONLY STRONG, SINEWY BRANCHES REMAIN FACING THE WIND."

MEDITATION

Your maturing body speaks the story of your life. Your victories and vulnerabilities are written in your unique form. Your body has been sculpted by your experience. Like the tree, you carry yourself strong and true, living to the best of your ability. You continue to reach for sunlight and energy while growing your wise roots deeply into the earth.

Celebrate your body's journey. Sing its song as you continue to dance along life's path.

~

"MY NEXT INHALE TINGLES WITH
LIFE. I REVEL IN BEING."

MEDITATION

Consider the miracle that you are alive on this incredible planet. Your living vibration is uniquely tangible. As you tap into the sensation of being vibrantly alive, you can find deep gratitude in every breath: exhaling living energy, and inhaling renewal.

~

ABOUT THE AUTHORS

BLESSING
OF THE COSMOS

May the

STRENGTH OF THE SUN
charge the aura of your being.

May the

SOFT LIGHT OF THE MOON
fill the Sea of Tranquility in your soul.

May you find

INSPIRATION IN THE STARS
like bright new ideas born from remnants of the past.

May the

SWIRLING DANCE OF OUR GALAXY
envelop you in the joy of belonging
in this magnificent universe.

About the Authors

Born and raised in New Orleans, Erik Krippner grew up with a po'boy in his hand and a song in his heart. As a boy, he spent his summers swimming, hiking, fishing, and sailing. After becoming an Eagle Scout, Erik dreamed of answering the call to "Go West, young man." He earned a Bachelor of Science degree in Forestry from Louisiana State University. Following his passion for adventure, Erik found his way to the mountains of the Pacific Northwest, his home to this day. After working in the forests of Oregon, Washington, Idaho, Alaska, Georgia, and Louisiana, Erik decided to focus his love of natural sciences on the study of human body through massage therapy.

Faye grew up in Oregon surrounded by family and old growth coastal forests. She spent many childhood weekends cross-country skiing, hunting for mushrooms, exploring coastal tide pools, and searching for crawdads in the Siuslaw River. Her love of books deepened when she became the editor of her high school and college's literary journals. Upon earning her Bachelor of Arts degree in Mathematics with honors from the Robert D. Clark Honors College at the University of Oregon, Faye became a technical writer and web developer. The whisper of a deeper purpose ignited her to study massage, where she met Erik.

Erik and Faye became friends in massage school at the East West College of the Healing Arts, in Portland, Oregon. In 2003, they founded Aqua Terra Massage, a therapeutic massage studio for friends and couples. Since then, they have practiced therapeutic massage together, side by side. They have spent years immersed in the study of massage, serving thousands of clients.

Faye and Erik have spent years exploring and writing about our beautiful world. They have sailed the blue waters of Fiji's Koro Sea, kayaked New Zealand's Marlborough Sound, and stargazed among the giraffes and elephants in Botswana. They have hiked the Appalachian Trail and paddled the tidally-influenced Columbia River in the Pacific Northwest. They have seen orca whales swim right under their kayaks, locked eyes with wild lions, and played hide-and-seek with an octopus. They have hiked thousands of miles together, kayaked and sailed hundreds, and spent countless evenings camping under the stars.

With a commitment to bringing more love and kindness to this beautiful world, we offer this book to you.

www.aquaterramassage.com